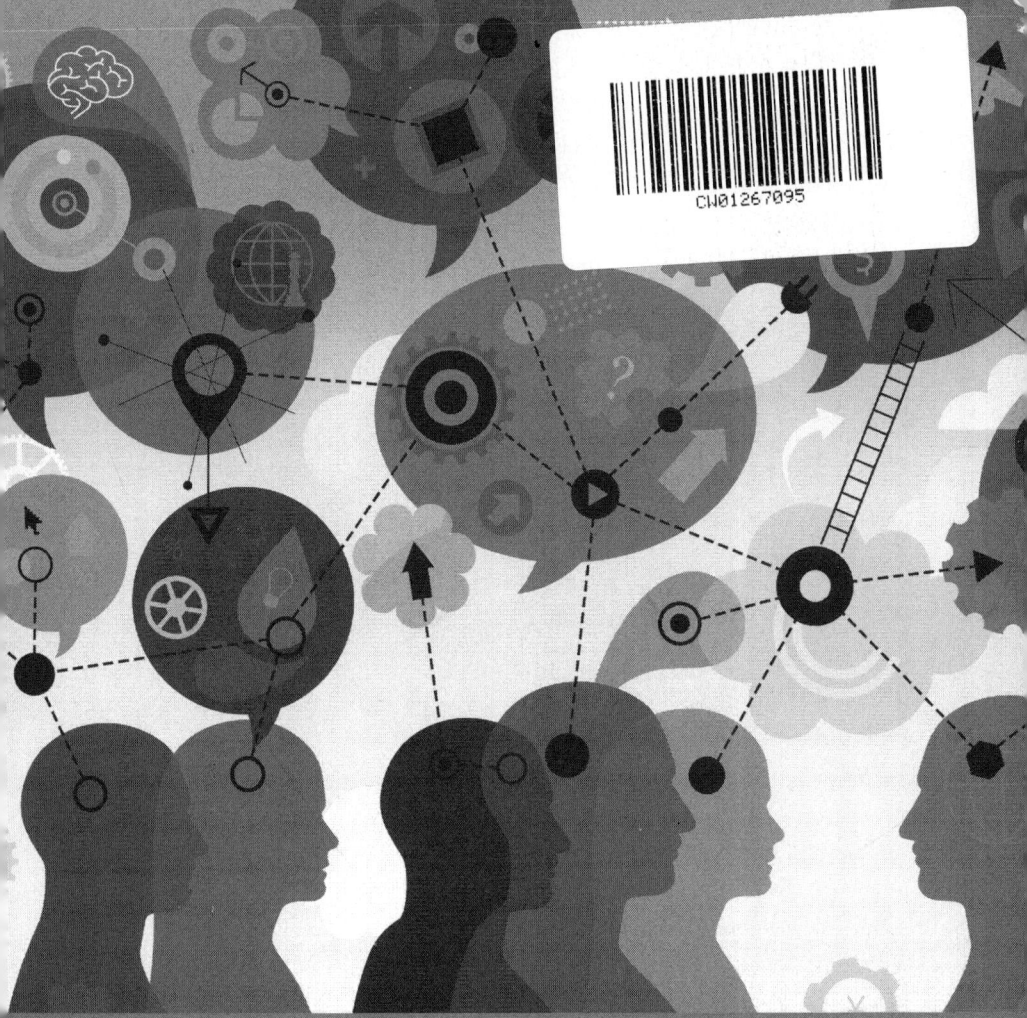

Applying Person-centred Care in Mental Health

A guide to values-based practice

By Wendy Hawksworth

Applying Person-centred Care in Mental Health
A guide to values-based practice

© Wendy Hawksworth 2016

The author has asserted her rights in accordance with the Copyright, Designs and Patents Act (1988) to be identified as the author of this work.

Published by:
Pavilion Publishing and Media Ltd
Rayford House
School Road
Hove
East Sussex
BN3 5HX
Tel: 01273 434 943
Fax: 01273 227 308
Email: info@pavpub.com

Published 2016 and 2017.

All rights reserved. No part of this publication may be reproduced, stored in a retrieval system, or transmitted in any form or by any means, electronic, mechanical, photocopying, recording or otherwise, without prior permission in writing of the publisher and the copyright owners.

A catalogue record for this book is available from the British Library.

ISBN: 978-1-911028-08-6
EPUB ISBN: 978-1-911028-33-8
EPDF ISBN: 978-1-911028-34-5
MOBI ISBN: 978-1-911028-35-2

Pavilion is the leading training and development provider and publisher in the health, social care and allied fields, providing a range of innovative training solutions underpinned by sound research and professional values. We aim to put our customers first, through excellent customer service and value.

Author: Wendy Hawksworth
Production editor: Ruth Chalmers, Pavilion Publishing and Media Ltd
Cover design: Emma Dawe, Pavilion Publishing and Media Ltd
Layout design: Phil Morash, Pavilion Publishing and Media Ltd
Printing: CMP Digital Print Solutions

Contents

About the author 2

Introduction 3

Section 1: The importance of working with values to provide person-centred care 9

Section 2: The importance of values for the person living with a mental illness – a historical perspective 15

Section 3: The importance of including all values relevant to the person 21

Section 4: How to stay connected with the person when there is a conflict of values 29

Section 5: How to stay connected with the person by being aware of different responses to values 37

Section 6: How to manage your values to keep the person central......45

Additional resources...53

Appendix..54

About the author

Wendy Hawksworth is a mental health nurse who works as a nurse educator in Brisbane. She has worked extensively with people with mental illness in the United Kingdom, New Zealand and Australia. She has wide experience in developing and delivering education and holds an MA in philosophy and psychiatry.

Wendy has presented at international conferences, is a member of the World Psychiatric Association (humanities section) and has co-authored a book chapter on values-based practice in multidisciplinary teams. She holds an adjunct lecturer title with the University of Queensland.

Introduction

Who is it for?
This guide is for staff working with people with a mental illness. Its focus is on inpatient units, however it also applies to staff working in the community. It provides a broad understanding of values-based practice. It is not exhaustive and hopefully not too directive, allowing you space to develop understanding from your experience. It can be used as a standalone document or to complement the skill-based training of VBP in the training pack that goes with this guide: *Applying Values-based Practice for People Experiencing Psychosis: A training pack for inpatient settings* (Hawksworth, 2016).

What is this guide based on?
This is a guide to providing person-centred care through a values-based approach. It is not about doing anything extra nor is it about therapy. It is about doing the work of being a mental health practitioner but doing it in a different way; a way that is inclusive of the patients' perspective, that is collaborative and based on engagement and respect. I use the terms 'mental illness' and 'patient' but also the term 'person', juxtaposing the medical language of patient with the ordinary language of person. This may feel awkward and at times uncomfortable, particularly when it relates to a hospital setting. Yet changing language can have a profound effect. Embracing new language and ways of explaining experiences to open up a space for the person's voice outside of their medical condition can allow new ways of thinking that bring to light new understandings, opportunities and ways of working.

As a concept, person-centred care is about keeping the person central to all care decisions. The Health Foundation (2014) has identified four principles of person-centred care:

1. Affording people dignity, compassion and respect.
2. Offering co-ordinated care, support or treatment.
3. Offering personalised care, support or treatment.
4. Supporting people to recognise and develop their own strengths and abilities to enable them to live an independent and fulfilling life.

It is clear from these principles that person-centred care is quite a shift in the traditional authoritarian and paternalistic approaches to care. The concept of 'clinician knows best' has changed to 'patient knows as well'. This is not patient from an illness only perspective but from the perspective of a person who is an expert on knowing what works for them in their lives, broader than just a patient. Collaborative approaches centred on the patients' values (their needs, wishes and desires at the time) ensure their personal perspective is included.

One of the challenges of person-centred care is to maintain the essence of the patient's perspective and ensure it is central to clinical decisions. This can be difficult for services when their values are misaligned with what the service and society deems as important for them. In a busy mental health service this may go unnoticed and values unexamined. This may lead to an assumption of inclusion and person-centred care. Examining the situation to determine whose values are being heard and whose are not so there is equal attention given to all, is an essential part of providing person-centered care. Being able to analyse the situation to differentiate between facts and values, and bring to light impasses based on dominant values, clears a space to consider the patient's perspective. Supporting their values being included, even when these may be different to the values of the dominant clinical group, is a way to practice person-centred care.

Values-based practice (VBP) provides a guide to how to do this. VBP supports the process of working through different values in particular situations. It was developed by K.W.M Fulford, who defines it as:

'The theory and skills base for effective healthcare decision making where different (and hence potentially conflicting) values are in play.'
(Woodbridge & Fulford, 2004)

This guide is about working with diverse values; that is the obvious (and heavily scrutinised), different values that the patient may bring when they become part of the service, and the not so obvious (more accepted), different values that the clinician brings as part of the service. Both contested and accepted, different and agreed values are questioned according to the perspective of the patient.

In order to provide collaborative care, the clinical relationship needs to be one based on trust and respect. Engagement and communication skills of VBP are based on a tolerance for the different values of the patient, rather than consensus of values. In this way, the fundamental concepts of person-centred care that rely on engagement are enabled. Tolerating different values of the person, even within restrictions that are placed upon them (i.e. they are on a section of the Mental Health Act) and exposing and challenging dominant values that exclude their personal perspective provides a space to do this. Empathising with a patient's perspective provides the means to do this.

As you go through the guide you will be exposed to both historical and present day practices that have shaped and continue to shape the way care is provided. Prioritising some values over others has resulted in inequalities and abuse. Past experiences can be shocking and lead us to question how this could have occurred, yet we are just as likely to have this concern today, derived from inequalities in practice. One way of tempering inequalities is to expose knowledge based on dominant values that take on a fact-like status, and which then lead to assumptions within practice that put the voice of staff over patients'. These value differences may challenge different meanings that are being considered in each situation, for example the concepts of risk, control and personal choice.

Perceived risks influence routines and decisions around what is or is not allowed. Keeping the patient from leaving the unit may be perceived by the clinician as the safest option, yet for the patient this decision may result in frustrations and behaviours that increase their risk of having medication forced on them or having to go to seclusion. Another example is where the clinician's perceived risk of not taking medication means that the patient will not improve, yet the patient may feel that it is taking medication that is making them unwell. This may be due to the side effects of the medication, which is a different concept of 'unwellness' than the clinician has. People (including people who use services and mental health professionals) are often self-contradictory and assumptions shouldn't be made that value statements are consistent (although personal values maybe). For example, a statement often made by professionals providing mental health care is a claim that they are giving people choice and control over their care (this is seen in the values statements of services and strategies) but this is equally what many people who use services say is taken away from them when they come into direct contact with mental health professionals.

Clearly this is a complex area, however VBP provides a guide to working across these differences by maintaining choice and participation rather than using coercion and control.

There is a 10 principle decision making framework that guides and enables clinicians to reflect on clinical decisions (see Appendix).

These are weaved throughout the guide as the various aspects of engagement and clinical decisions are considered. It examines values used in clinical practice, how they present in different situations and how they influence clinical decisions. It will assist you to critique and monitor your practice in order to maintain best care according to the patient's perspective. By listening first to the person living with the experience and making decisions inclusive of their perspective, it ensures respect by the inclusion of their values. One of the concerns from clinicians of VBP is that it asks them to give away their learnt knowledge. This is certainly not the case and as you go through the guide you will see how the 'professional' /scientific knowledge and the knowledge of the person living with the experience are considered together. In this way it provides clinicians with a broader approach from which to base decisions, thereby enriching rather than detracting from clinical knowledge.

How to work with values from a person-centred perspective

In order to be person-centred we need to be mindful of the way values are used and the way they influence decisions of care. The 'how to' of VBP involves a series of reflective questions that are formed around four practice skills of awareness, reasoning, knowledge and communication.

In order to work from a values-based perspective you need to stop and think about the decision you are making, leaving your values to one side to engage with the person in your care. The relevant skills are:

1: Awareness
Bringing to awareness the values that are influencing your decisions. Reflecting in the moment to consider decisions through questions such as: whose values are influencing my thoughts at this time? Whose values are being given priority? Am I aware of all the values important to the patient at this time?

2: Reasoning
How informed is my reasoning? Is my reasoning emotionally driven or is it derived from a place of understanding? Am I presuming and interpreting using judgements and inferences without being truly informed?

3: Knowledge

How inclusive is my knowledge base? Is there other information that may help? Is my knowledge base being influenced by my personal values, the values of the organisation or my professional values?

4: Communication

Is my communication approach inclusive, sensitive, respectful and informed according to the patient's identified needs at this time?

Using these four points to reflect on the scenarios within this guide will provide you with the practice to then apply within the clinical area as different scenarios take shape.

Section 1: The importance of working with values to provide person-centred care

Skill: awareness

What are values?

Let us start at the beginning of our journey by considering values. What are they? Values do not lend themselves to one clear definition. They comprise many different beliefs and cultural norms. Their composition is broad. Fulford says:

'Values come in many different varieties: epistemic aesthetic and prudential as well as moral and ethical; they take different logical forms (e.g. needs, wishes, desires); they have many origins (e.g. personal, professional, cultural) and they have a rich grammar (encompassing nouns, verbs, adverbs).'
(Fulford, 2004, p208)

Basically, values reflect anything that is valued. That is, anything important that is valued by an organisation, society, person or profession. Our personal values make us the unique human beings that we are. They help us consider what is right and wrong and include our personal desires and likes and dislikes.

Values are what we believe is good or bad, wrong or right; they are about the choices we make and influence the way we see the world and the things we do.

Facts provide an objective truth, values provide a subjective truth

Values are a matter of personal preference. My personal preference is to favour living in the countryside. The reason for this is I like the space and being amongst nature. This is what I value. You may hold different values and prefer to live closer to the city valuing an easy commute to work or access to the city infrastructure. Both preferences are about individual values and neither one is right or wrong, only different. On the other hand it is a fact that I am writing this guide on a computer. If you disputed this, you would be wrong. So there is a certain objective truth about facts whereas there is a subjective truth about values. In the busyness of the mental health service the patient's subjective truth can be overlooked resulting in them being left out of their care decisions. This is particularly the case where the meaning of their subjective truth is deemed irrational due to their mental illness. This can stand in contrast to clinician's subjective truth that can be seen as fact. It is important that we monitor the basis of our beliefs and check in with the patient to avoid making assumptions that isolate their perspective. Making clinical decisions that are inclusive of the patients' values ensures that their subjective truth is considered, thereby maintaining a person-centred approach.

> **Thinking activity:**
> What do you consider values to be? Jot down some responses. Can you identify clusters of values which have common elements?

Benefit of engaging with all values

The primary benefit of working with values is that it empowers the patient to have a voice broader then a medical view. The person is given permission to have a legitimate place in clinical conversations and practices which allows them to be involved in their care. For the clinician, becoming aware of the patient's values provides a space to re-focus on the human aspects of working in mental health and gives opportunities to care. These mutually beneficial aspects of VBP of being cared about and caring about, are shared between the patient and the clinician. Working from a values-based perspective will support you in choosing clinical decisions that are person-centred, enriching your experience of being part of the patients' unique care and their experience of having a part in how their care is provided.

Shared perspectives of working with values

Benefits of working with values	Drawback of not working with values
Working with values benefits both patients and staff by opening up a space for aspects of the patient to become known, in addition to a medical perspective. In this way, it adds to clinical knowledge and supports person-centred care.	Not including all values can lead to practices that are rigid and institutional. These become habits of practice derived from generalised applications according to the way things have always been done, rather than in response to individual needs.
Working with values benefits both patients and staff by including all values that play a part in the situation, thereby providing a collaborative approach that involves carers, significant others and the multidisciplinary team.	Not including all values may limit access to essential knowledge. It can lead to one type of knowledge dominating. It can lead to both staff and patients feeling unfulfilled. Staff may feel dissatisfied with work; patients may feel dissatisfied with treatment.
Working with values benefits both staff and patients by providing a service that is meaningful and responsive, reducing the need for control and coercion.	Not including all values can lead to both staff and patients being at risk. Aggression and violent situations fuelled by invalidation can be tempered by considering values.
There may be times when the person is at risk to themselves or others and direct control needs to be exercised. This does not however preclude engaging with values. Being aware of values and keeping the process of values engagement active in different situations means challenges are not ignored but worked through.	

Why it is necessary to include values to provide an ethical approach?

The work of delivering healthcare is framed according to fixed ethical codes and standards. These ethically based principles guide clinicians to make decisions that are reasoned and morally sound. No matter what profession you work within e.g. occupational therapy, nursing or social work, you will be accountable for your practice, according to governing ethical standards. These provide a top-down generic approach to ethical care that goes across healthcare services. However the work of delivering healthcare is also influenced by the needs of the patient. Unlike principles, these needs are variable and individual. They are derived from a bottom-up approach according to their desires at the time.

These two ethical guides of principles and personal perspectives need to be considered together to ensure ethical care reflects the variables of the individual. The following explains how these two areas of ethics work.

Top-down principle-based approach

In modern healthcare we are subject to the big values questions, such as patients' rights to self-determination, capacity to make informed decisions and the right to take one's own life. These are the big ethical questions; the big ticket items determined through ethical principles that advise on the best approach. Beauchamp and Childress (1994) have identified four ethical principles that are important in healthcare:

- Beneficence – doing good as far as possible.
- Non-maleficence – minimising or preventing harm.
- Justice – fairness and equal access to care.
- Autonomy – respect for individual self-determination.

These drive professional values. They sit within codes of practice and standards of care to guide the clinician to make the best decision.

Bottom-up values-based approach

Our decisions are also influenced by all the little ticket items that are particular to values. These may be considered little tickets items in that they are not the generic, big questions, however this doesn't mean they are not big items for the person and can make a profound difference to their well-being. In this case, advice about what is the best approach comes from the individuals involved in the situation at the time. Patients' values are central, but the values of friends, family, carers and clinicians may also be relevant in assisting the patient. Decisions are made according to the different values of the people involved. Medical knowledge is also considered as it also plays a part in decision making.

The following provides a clinical example.

> **Case example: The interplay between a top-down and bottom-up approach**
>
> Sonia is a 54-year-old lady who has been admitted to the mental health unit for the first time. She has a long history of mental illness but is not known to the service. She was referred by her son Damien who thought that his mum needed to see someone as she had stopped eating. She was admitted to the ward looking tired and dishevelled. She was unclear why she needed to be in a mental health unit. She spent the early days of her admission alone in her bedroom reluctant to talk about her situation and refusing to eat. She said all the food had been poisoned. The admitting doctor prescribed antidepressants.
>
> Sonia stayed in her room. Her son brought meals he knew she would like which she ate in her room.

- Ethical principles tell us what we need to do.
- Sonia's values tell us how to do it.
- Damien's values help us to do it.
- Doctor's knowledge provides a medical perspective.

Ethical principles	What needs to happen
Beneficence.	Need to help her well-being.
Non-maleficence.	Need to act to avoid harm.
Justice.	Need to ensure she receives appropriate healthcare.
Autonomy.	Need to support her independence.

Section 1: The importance of working with values to provide person-centred care

Sonia's values	How to do it
Hospital food is poisoned.	Not all food is poisoned; she will eat food brought in by her son.
Does not trust the staff.	Prefers some staff over others – allocate these staff.
Does not care if she lives or dies.	Just wants to be left alone – respect privacy.
Does not trust other people.	Will listen to her son – include son in care plan.
Feels unsafe in hospital.	Feels safer in her room – support care in her room.

Damien's values	Helping us to do it
Want to see his mum get back to her old self.	Damien talks to mum and reassures her that she will get back to her old self again.
Wants his mum to eat.	Brings food in for his mum.
Respects the medical opinion.	Talks to the doctors about his mum's wishes and advises on what will help her.
Wants to be involved in his mum's care.	Takes time off work to be with his mum.

Doctor's medical knowledge	Providing evidence-based practice
Completes investigations and screens to diagnose and treat Sonia's condition.	Completes regular mental state examinations and mental health assessments.
Treats and monitors Sonia's symptoms.	Prescribes anti-depressants and anti-psychotics.
Includes Sonia in information about her medical condition.	Talks to Sonia about her medication and her medical condition.
Ensures her physical health needs are met.	Investigates and treats Sonia's physical health.

Thinking activity:
What do you notice about the different perspectives?
How would decisions be made if we only considered principles?

Section 2: The importance of values for the person living with a mental illness – a historical perspective

Skill: awareness

Case example: Grace's story

'My name is Grace. I am a 20-year-old student nurse training to be a mental health nurse in a large 1,000 bed mental hospital on the outskirts of the city.

I am in my second year of training. There are 16 nurses in our year. Most of us live in the nurse's home which is on site. The hospital is situated in a small village. There is a bus into town which runs once per hour. There is a staff canteen and staff social club on site.

As a student, I go to some of the wards which are deemed training wards but some I don't go to. I spend three months on each ward. I am out for six months and then will be back in school for three weeks. The nursing school is on site.

The year is 1979 and I am working in a 23-bed female ward. I am here for three months.

This is an example of my day shift:

I arrive on the ward at 7am and we have a handover from the night staff. The first job is to get the patients up and give them their breakfast. The night staff get some of the patients up and we get the others up. The patients are in two large dormitories. It is a female-only ward. They have a bed with a wardrobe alongside, separating one bed from the next. We choose what the patient will be wearing for the day and help them to get dressed. The clothes come from the laundry. We sort the clothes out every afternoon. It's usually a random choice of what will fit who. Sometimes the choice is not that good and when we get them dressed in a morning the dress can be too tight or a bit short for them. If we run short we borrow from someone else's wardrobe.

Continued

Case example: Grace's story Continued

We escort them to the day room where they sit in a soft chair or take them straight into the dining room to wait for breakfast.

At 8:30am breakfast arrives. It is sent down from the kitchen already prepared. It is the same every day: porridge and scrambled eggs and beans. It is the ward sister's job to dish the food out. The night staff have laid the tables, so we move the patients into the dining room and give them their breakfast.

When this has finished, they go back to the day room. Some of them go to the industrial therapy unit which is about a 10 minute walk on the other side of the hospital. One of the staff will go with them whilst the others stay and make beds, shower people as required and tidy the living area. Morning medications are dispensed from a mobile trolley in the day room. Cigarettes are given to the patients on an hourly basis.

At 10:30am we break for morning tea. We make the tea for the patients. We put the milk in the tea pot because it is easier. Whilst they are having their morning tea we also have ours. On this ward the nurse makes coffee made with milk for us which is just lovely.

Lunch time is midday. Again the food is nice and soft so the patients won't choke. After lunch they sit in the day room. If it is a nice day they may sit outside on the balcony. Martha is one of the more capable patients who helps give the tea out. She can be a bit bossy with the other patients and we have to keep her in check.

Lunch time medication is given from the medication trolley in the dining room whilst the patients are having their lunch. Because I am a student, I can't dispense it on my own so I work as the runner giving it to the patients when the sister has dispensed it. The main medications are chlorpromazine and promazine. These tend to be given in liquid form so the sister can adjust the dose and give more if she thinks the patient needs it.

Topical medications are used sometimes to rub into patients because they have skin patches either on their head or knees from the continual movement.

We write the notes at 2:30 pm and the afternoon staff come on duty.'

Doing to the person: when values are not heard

Historically people with mental illness were seen as having little to contribute to society. As a result, large numbers of people were treated in isolated institutions far away from the rest society. These institutions cared for people with mental illness. People were housed and looked after, however there was something fundamental that was missing and that was the connection with their values. Unlike Grace the nurse, the patients had no acknowledged story.

Patients lived, socialised, worked, were treated, died and were buried in the institutions. Patients worked within the institutions; maybe on the farm, industrial therapy unit or in the laundry. Like the patients, staff also worked and lived within the institutions. There were hospital houses for staff, a staff canteen, schools of nursing on site and a staff social club. Staff work was centred on set routines that enabled them to complete tasks with the largest number of patients. These daily routines were applied to groups of patients at any one time. Routine shower times, routine meal times and routine bed times were all part of the social infrastructure that enabled the wheels of the institution to turn.

Sitting behind the growth of these institutions was a dominant medical model. The grouping together of people in this way advantaged the profession of psychiatry by enabling new treatments to be tried and tested. It also provided opportunities to examine behaviours from which psychiatry could forge its profession.

This medical approach reflected the thinking of the time which was based on medical paternalism, where decisions were made on behalf of the patient according to what was deemed to be best for them. This approach was particularly oppressive in psychiatry because of the use of involuntary treatment. Unlike general health, patients in institutions had no options to determine their treatment. This led to a dominant autocratic approach of psychiatry that supported supremacy of one set of values over another. Practices within institutions reflected this imbalance of values.

The system operated in a way that was blind to the patients' values. There was no values disagreement, because there was no other voice heard. Patients were not consulted and staff made decisions according to the parameters of set routines. Routines set the pace and the whole process ticked over like clockwork. Decisions were straightforward and life within the institutions was uncomplicated. Things were pretty straightforward, decisions were easy and alternative values were seldom expressed.

> **Thinking activity:**
> Think about Grace's story and the relationship of values and the de-humanising of the person. When we do not consider the patient's values, there is a distancing from the human connection. This can and has in the past led to a slippery slope into abuse and neglect.

When values are repressed: the risk of not being heard

Deegan (1992) wrote about a cycle of disempowerment where invalidation of the person led to a self-perpetuating state of chronicity.

The central attitudinal barrier
People with psychiatric disabilities cannot be self-determining because to be mentally ill means to have lost the capacity for sound reasoning. It means one is irrational and 'crazy'. Thus all of the thoughts, choices, expressions etc. of persons who have been diagnosed with mental illness can be ignored.

The system takes control
Therefore professionals within the organisation must take responsibility for us.

LEARNED HELPLESSNESS

The prophecy is fulfilled
As we become experts in being helpless patients the central barrier is reinforced.

Figure 2.1 The cycle of disempowerment and despair. Reprinted with permission from Deegan P (1992) The independent living movement and people with psychiatric disabilities: taking back control over our own lives. *Psychosocial Rehabilitation Journal* **15** (3) 12.

In this situation there was little option for change and institutions practised in this way for more than 100 years.

During this time the person was seen as the sum total of their illness, rather than an individual. Schizophrenia was termed *dementia praecox*, that is, premature dementia. It was seen as a chronic disease that was unremitting, leading to progressive deterioration and early death.

There was a focus on physical treatments such as lobotomies, deep insulin therapy and electric convulsive therapy (ECT). ECT is the only physical therapy that continues today. The following table highlights these perceptions.

Concept	Consequence
Mental illness was seen as abnormal.	Derogatory terms were used to describe people: nutter, psycho, schizo, crazy, lunatic etc.
The cause was derived from a physical problem yet to be found.	Treated in social isolation.
Era of medical paternalism where the doctor knew best.	Patient voice not heard.
Person was seen as the sum total of their illness.	Individual needs outside the parameters of the illness were not heard.
Generalised approaches.	Greatest good to the greatest number.
Generalisable criteria.	Routines of practice and treatment.

Section 3: The importance of including all values relevant to the person

Skill: reasoning

In the last section we looked at how some institutional practices could invalidate the person due to an imbalance between dominant medical values and patient values. During the era of institutional care, treatment was particularly oppressive. There has however, over time, been an increase in the voice of the patient through the recovery movement and the work of mental health charities such as SANE, Mental Health Foundation and Rethink Mental Illness. These groups have contributed to changing public perception of psychiatry. Yet bringing person-centred practice change into inpatient units continues to be a significant challenge. Although we have moved on from institutional settings, the care within acute wards often includes practices that invalidate the person. This specific issue has been discussed in depth in Faulkner (2005).

Today this issue is not so much under an umbrella of medical paternalism but under an umbrella of perceived risk. Today we have moved away from treating people in institutions:

- People are treated in psychiatric units attached to general hospitals.
- Psychiatry has included a bio-psychosocial, spiritual and cultural approach to enhance the medical view.
- Where possible people live in society and are treated in the community.

The move to general hospitals has aligned mental illness with physical illness. There was a belief that this would reduce the stigma associated with having a mental illness. Yet this has proved difficult. One of the reasons for this may be the difference in values. Values aligned with physical illness tend to be straightforward and agreed, whereas values in mental health are more diverse and not necessarily in keeping with what is considered acceptable behaviour. The person who is psychotic may behave in ways that are difficult to comprehend compared to the behaviour of patients with a physical illness. Behaviour that is difficult to understand and seems irrational can be seen as threatening or as a nuisance that needs to be controlled. Attempts to control behaviour have over time resulted in increasing laws and restrictions being applied to patients.

The expected autonomy from living in the community post de-institutionalisation has become conditional upon behaving in certain ways. No longer is the person locked away out of sight and mind but they are in full view with the opinion of society judging their worth and need for treatment.

The following exercise will allow you to start to consider the values-laden nature of mental health and the influence this has on our reasoning.

Complete the following to compare the different ways of reasoning in these two scenarios.

Values laden nature of mental health: a comparison with physical illness

The story of Tania: two alternative scenarios

1. Tania is a 35-year-old woman living in a suburb of Brisbane. Tania has no children. One day during the winter of 2013 Tania slipped on some water on her stairs and smashed her leg into the wall. The neighbours heard her shouting for help. The emergency services were called and she ended up being taken to hospital. Tania was diagnosed as having fractured both the tibia and fibula of her left leg.

2. Tania is a 35-year-old woman living in a suburb of Brisbane. Tania has no children. One day during the winter of 2013 Tania knocked on the neighbour's door demanding that they stop talking about her. The emergency services were called and she was taken to hospital. Tania was diagnosed with schizophrenia.

What springs to mind as you consider the two scenarios?

Consider each question in turn and respond.

1: Cause and effect
What is the cause of Tania's broken leg?

What is the cause of Tania's schizophrenia?

2: The process of hospitalisation
What part do you think Tania played in the process of getting to hospital?

Tania's role was different in the two scenarios… what do you consider are these differences?

The neighbour had involvement in both of the scenarios but in a different way. What is this difference?

What is the different involvement of the emergency services in each scenario?

Section 3: The importance of including all values relevant to the person

What are the consequences for Tania in the two scenarios? _____
_____
_____
_____

3: Social effects on illness
What may be the impact of the social situation on Tania?
_____
_____
_____

From a general health perspective? _____
_____
_____
_____

From a mental health perspective?
_____
_____
_____

4: Cultural effects on illness
Imagine that Tania was living in Africa at the time.

Would this affect the concept of bodily illness? Would it affect her diagnosis of a fractured tibia and fibula?
_____
_____
_____

Would this affect the concept of mental illness? Would it affect her diagnosis of schizophrenia? _____
_____
_____

What is the reason for this difference? _____
_____
_____
_____

5: Different ways of knowing

How is the diagnosis of a fractured tibia and fibula known? What are the mechanisms for assessment? _____
_____
_____

How is the diagnosis of schizophrenia known? What are the mechanisms for assessment? _____
_____
_____

6: Consider judgements

What judgements are made about a person with a broken leg? Write down words that come to mind that may reflect general consensus around the person who has a broken leg. _____
_____
_____
_____

What are the judgements made about a person with schizophrenia? Write down words that come to mind that may reflect general consensus around the person living with schizophrenia. _____
_____
_____
_____

Consider the reason for this. _____
_____
_____
_____

What if rather than a broken leg Tania had diabetes?
_____
_____
_____

What if rather than schizophrenia Tania had depression?

_____
_____
_____

> **Thinking activity:**
> Jot down a list of points around reasoning that you could be aware of when you are making clinical person-centred decisions.

How to balance reasoning

The dominant risk agenda has largely resulted in values being out of balance. Inpatient units have increasingly focused on control and containment at the expense of personal autonomy. This has fed into a medical approach based on problem and deficits. Moving away from a culture based on risk requires a move that empowers patients to make informed decisions.

The challenge is how to balance the two agendas of risk management and patient autonomy, as clinical situations play out on a daily basis.

Risk: self and/or others	Autonomy: patient values
Doctor knows best.	Patients' right to steer their own care.
Treatment enforced.	Patients' right to determine their own treatment.
Legal aspect of enforcing treatment.	Patients' human rights.
Response to social situation.	Response to patient wishes.
Practices of coercion and control.	Patients' right to self-determination.
Practice based on deficits and problems.	Patient is seen as more than their illness.
Risk averse.	Patients' right to take risks.

The above table highlights the differences between risk management-based control and patient autonomy. Neither one of these approaches are necessarily wrong, however exclusive use of either one is a potential problem. A dominant risk management approach can lose sight of the patient as a person, whereas a dominant person-centred perspective can lose sight of the medical view. The following provides examples of this from the perspective of Mary. Mary's health and care decisions reflect two very different views. Where the perceived risk is high her behaviour is considered to be due to her mental illness. She is described through this and care decisions are made accordingly. Where the perceived risk is low her behaviour is understood in a very ordinary non-medical way. Terms reflect a citizen's rights perspective.

Case example: Mary

Mary is a 56-year-old lady who is in the inpatient unit. She has been on the ward for two weeks. She spends time in her room and chooses not to be involved in ward activities. Staff consider their role as therapeutic guests. This is where the person's mental health condition is not considered. Staff are there as 'guests' to take the lead from the person. Mary's response is to tell them to go away and leave her alone. They consider Mary's response as reflecting her choice without question.

Mary is a 56-year-old lady who is in the inpatient unit. She has been on the ward for two weeks. She spends time in her room and is non-compliant with ward activities. Her behaviour is seen as part of her illness. She is psychotic, hearing voices and is isolated and withdrawn. Treatment is enforced in order to address Mary's problems and deficits. Staff members are seen as medical experts.

Mary is seen as a mental illness	Mary is seen as a person with no mental illness
Behaviour viewed as isolated and withdrawn.	Expresses a desire to be alone.
Behaviour judged as being non-compliant.	Chooses not to be involved.
Behaviour seen as part of her pathology.	Would like to focus on her wishes and desires.
Focus on symptoms as a problem and deficit.	Doesn't have a problem with her symptoms.

There is clearly a distinct divide between both of these approaches. The medical only perspective is derived from judgments and interpretations. The person only perspective is considered in isolation of the impact of the mental illness on their behaviour. To balance these it is necessary to be mindful of not throwing the baby out with the bath water and neglecting the medical perspective, while tempering interpretations. Trying to understand the meaning of the behaviour for the person is one way of balancing these two perspectives. Meeting in the middle will require flexibility, trust and a more balanced approach to a dominant risk agenda.

A balanced approach: the interface between mental illness and individual choice

> Mary is a 56-year-old lady who is on the inpatient unit. She has been on the ward for two weeks. She spends time in her room because she is scared of being with other people. When she was first admitted, she witnessed one of the patients getting angry, security being called and alarms going off and people fighting. Since then she has stayed in her room. She hears voices which tell her to keep away from others. She wishes she could be discharged.

This approach brings in Mary's psychosis and the relationship between this with her experience of being in the unit. Rather than separating her psychosis from the situation they are understood together. This provides a reason for Mary's current behaviour and her wishes around this. With this information, person-centred clinical decisions can then be made that reflect Mary's particular situation broader than her mental illness.

Section 4: How to stay connected with the person when there is a conflict of values

Skills: awareness and reasoning

Reactions to conflict

Control and coercion are sometimes used to enforce compliance in situations where there are different values.

Here are some examples of shutting down different values when there is a values disagreement:

- Demanding the person takes their medication.
- Threatening that if they do not stop shouting they will go into the high dependency unit.
- Using seclusion to control emotions.
- Injecting the person against their will.
- Using long acting depot medication to enforce medication compliance.

The above practice examples are ones at the extreme end of the conflict line: the types of conflicts that demand attention. When this happens, the person is 'done to' and the conflict is managed by shutting down different values that are seen to be a problem. These examples are about enforcing treatment when engagement and negotiation have broken down. Maybe the situation was unavoidable and it was necessary to take control because the person's or another person's life was in immediate danger, but maybe it could have been avoided. VBP is about trying to find ways to avoid this situation.

Just because we are not hearing a different view does not mean that one does not exist

Values are dynamic and they present at different times in different situations. Working with the person's values throughout their stay in the inpatient unit is necessary to understand this dynamic.

To provide person-centred care, we need to be attuned to values. Values need to be considered not only at the end of the line of treatment when a situation erupts, but at the beginning and throughout the process. Effective treatment is about using values to work across all the practices that occur before we get to the end of the line – from admission to discharge, during communication and documentation, risk and mental health assessment, policies and procedures – in other words, in everything we do.

In order to work with the person before there is a clash of values, we need to link with values that are not noticed. Two types of values – implicit and explicit – are described below.

Implicit values

We use values all the time to make decisions without being consciously aware of them. The approach we take, the way we conduct ourselves, what we do and don't do are influenced by our values. They are really powerful, yet most of the time we are not aware of them. They are implicit. We tend to only notice them when we have to make a difficult decision and we weigh up what values are good and bad, right and wrong. When decisions are easy, our values are aligned and decisions run smoothly.

My decision to walk to the kitchen and get a cup of tea was driven by a physiological need to quench my thirst and also to get a caffeine fix. I could have opted for a cup of water or a coffee but I prefer the taste of tea. I prefer tea to the point of exerting effort and boiling the kettle, getting milk and making tea. My preference for tea motivated me to do this. This was a straight forward decision – it was easy. My values of liking a cup of tea influenced my behaviour which I acted on without being consciously aware of them. Unless we actively think about what was important for us around a decision, we just go along with it unaware of the values that underpin it.

In cases like this, our values and choices are aligned, making the decision easy and the values silent. This happens on a day-to-day basis, as our values drive us to make decisions that fit with what is important for us.

Explicit values

We become aware of values when we are faced with other values that are different to ours. These are explicit values.

The easiness of my decision to make a cup of tea may have been challenged if my daughter had drunk the last of the milk and I did not like tea without it. Not a particularly earth shattering situation, but one that would have been enough to affront my values when challenged. My desire for a cup of tea would have been subsumed by my daughter's desire for a glass of milk. My reaction would have depended on my state of mind at the time, the situation and the options for a solution. Maybe I had just finished a night shift and was tired, it was raining heavily and I did not have the car to go and buy more milk. This may have happened before and I had previously asked her not to drink the last of the milk. There are lots of reasons that can influence our reactions.

My reaction would be that my daughter was inconsiderate, selfish and did not consider her mum who had just come in from work. This would, however, be an ill-considered response derived from my values without knowing what my daughter's situation was. This would inflame rather than regulate the clash of values. It may have been that my daughter drank the milk because she was feeling ill and this helped her to feel better. But I was not aware of this, and jumped to conclusions according to my values. For me to consider both sides, I would have to put aside my values for a time and try to understand my daughter's situation by engaging with reason rather than emotion.

Emotional reactions in situations where there is a power differential such as this parent and child example can result in the use of control and even punishment to demand adherence. I may shout and tell her that she is to go to the shops and get some milk. In adult situations this behaviour may be mirrored when there is one group that is more vulnerable than the other.

A person who is in the psychiatric unit is one such example. Shutting down the values difference by power and control may lead to bullying or intimidation. In extreme cases this can lead to the use of control and coercion to demand obedience to different values.

What this looks like from a clinical perspective

Clinically, values between the patient and medical practitioners tend to run smoothly. This enables routines of practice such as set medication, set meal times and set visiting times. We house people in mixed wards, we place people we consider at risk under The Mental Health Act (1983), we interpret and judge behaviour according to set criteria determined from pre-determined categories.

This way of working is fine as long as this approach is supported by all concerned. Values are implicit and silent. We presume they are agreed, but there are many reasons in mental health why values may not be agreed. The patient may not believe they have a mental illness and would rather not be there. They may not be happy about being in a mixed ward. They may not like being nursed by male staff and may prefer to not take their medication. They may wish to leave the unit.

With patients from all walks of life, the values within a mental health unit are diverse. But these are not just individual preferences; they are cultural, ethical, spiritual and gender values as well. Joan prefers to be in a female-only ward and prefers female staff because of her history of sexual abuse. Robert prefers not to take his medication because of the side effects that affect his libido. Karl has been living on the streets for years and he finds it really difficult to be in the unit. Mary does not think she has a mental illness and should not be in the unit as in her culture, people are not locked away but are part of society.

Mental health units are alive with different values and potential for conflict. We are working from our set of values that may not necessarily be shared. It is important that we know what the patients' values are.

Thinking activity:
Do you consider the values of the patients in your care?
How are you including them in what you do?

Working with conflict by considering the person first

Ideally we would like to work with values before there is conflict. In order to do this, patients' values need to be known and included in clinical conversations.

Here are a couple of steps to start the process of knowing:

Step 1. Assume that values are part of the situation. Values are behind the particular response and are something that needs further exploration.

Step 2. Get to know what these values are.

Step 1: Assume that values are part of the situation

Balancing decisions

Fundamentally, mental illness does not stand on its own without a person. You cannot separate the person from the illness. Yet when the illness is considered in isolation of the person's perspective we are only working from part of the presentation. When medical values dominate, it is easy to make decisions that do not consider the values of the person. For example:

- Keeping the person on the Mental Health Act because they are hearing voices but not considering how they feel about hearing voices.

- Keeping the person on the Mental Health Act to give depot injections because they are refusing to take oral medication but not considering the reason why they are not taking their medication.

- Keeping the person on the Mental Health Act because they want to leave the unit without considering the reason why they want to leave.

Bringing the person into the equation

To bring the person to mind we need to connect with our shared humanness. We need to be able to see the situation from a human perspective that derives from a place of understanding, tolerance and compassion. Being able to empathise helps us to bring the person into the view.

When we omit to see the person's perspective in a conflict situation, we can react in very different ways. Whether we are open to the person's perspective or not depends on how we see the reason for the conflict:

- If we see the primary cause of conflict as a chemical condition that requires medication, then the use of control to enforce medication may be justified (for example the person who has a drug induced psychosis).

- If we see the primary cause of conflict as a reaction to a frustrating situation then finding out about it and trying to work something out around it may be justified.

Thinking activity:
Consider times when you hear reference to a person's behaviour that is not based on understanding the situation. What are the words that are used to explain this?

Step 2: Get to know what these values are

Case example: Michael

With this in mind complete the following activity:

Michael has been admitted to the unit on a forensic order following a conviction for serious violence. He had stopped taking his anti-psychotic medication some months before admission and had been erratically using alcohol and street drugs. The deterioration in his mental state had been accompanied by increasing aggression – a direct result of psychotic experience. On the ward, Michael has apparently resumed taking his medication, but his symptoms have not been completely resolved.

It is 8am and Michael is in the dining room for breakfast. He appears to be responding to voices and has started to shout at other patients across the table.

You are the nurse in charge.

The junior nurse asks you to call security to take Michael to his room to give him an injection.

There are three questions that you need to ask the junior nurse to help you decide what to do.

What are they?

Avoiding control by considering the person's perspective

Considering the person's perspective allows us to regulate our response. Rather than using medication and seclusion, maybe we need to find a place to talk about the situation and find out what is going on for the person. Trying to understand the conflict as a human reaction which may contribute to the person's chemical condition allows us to start from a place of being curious about their values.

> **Thinking activity:**
> What questions could you ask the person who does not want their medication, considering their potentially different values?

Words that shut down connecting with the person:
- Demanding.
- Isolative.
- Insightless.
- Non-compliant.
- Irritable.
- Escalating.
- Manipulative.
- Splitting.
- Attention seeking.
- Self-defeating.
- Oppositional.
- Passive aggressive.

Actions that shut out the person's values:
- Not being inclusive.
- Speaking down to the person.
- Not sharing knowledge and expectations.
- Ignoring the person.

- 'Doing' to the person without consultation.
- Speaking to the person like a child.
- Using harsh words.
- Using language that is not clear.
- Viewing the person negatively by seeing only the problem.
- Shouting.
- Being unfair by using one rule for one person and another for others.
- Not explaining what the problem is.
- Being inflexible to the individual's needs.
- Talking over the person.

Tips to ensure the patient's perspective is heard:
- Respect the other person.
- Accept that their values may be different.
- Get to know your patient and what is important for them.
- Know what the patient's values are and make them central to your plan.
- Talk about and include the patient's values in the multidisciplinary team review.
- Check in with your understanding.
- Be dynamic, flexible and inclusive.
- Consider your pre-judgements.
- Leave your medical knowledge to one side to engage with the person's perspective.
- Be curious and inquisitive.

Section 5: How to stay connected with the person by being aware of different responses to values

Skills: awareness, reasoning and communication

Being aware of different responses to values

This section is about values being heard. It examines the ones that do not outwardly show themselves and the responses we have to them that disable them from being heard. These are the values that we take for granted, are OK, yet we do not really know about. These are the ones that, when we do not engage with them, we inadvertently shut them down and shut the person off. I will introduce you to the ways this is done and ask you to consider them through the story of Paul. We will start with Paul's story.

> **Case example: Paul**
>
> Paul is a 26-year-old man who has recently been admitted to the mental health unit.
>
> Music is a large part of Paul's life. He plays guitar and writes songs. Since his admission he has lost his accommodation and has brought all that he owns on to the unit. This is not a lot: one laundry bag of clothes and one guitar. Paul spends all day playing his guitar.
>
> *Continued*

> *Case example: Paul continued*
>
> He does not have a regular place to live. His mum and dad are estranged and live in different parts of the country. He has not seen them for about three years and has lost touch with them. He has a brother Sif who has been supportive but Paul prefers to be around his friends. They usually let him hang out with them at their place, sleeping on couches and decks wherever he can.
>
> He was admitted to the mental health unit under the Mental Health Act, being brought in by the police in handcuffs and placed in the high dependency unit. Paul does not have much memory of what brought this on and is not sure why he should be in the mental health unit. He believes he has special powers and that he would be better using his powers outside the unit to influence the course of world events rather than being locked up. Being in the unit is holding him back from doing this. He does not agree that he needs to be there or that his thinking is problematic. He takes his medication because he is made to and has in the past been given injections when he chooses not to. He really does not like injections; the thought of something eating away inside destroying his soul makes him feel scared. His powers are really important for him and he needs to keep in touch with them. He talks to his friends about it when they visit. He would like to continue to use his powers in the unit but does not talk to the staff about it because he does not trust them. He tries to get around this by spending time alone in his room when he connects with his spiritual self and feels in a space that allows him to do this. He connects spiritually by chanting. He shares a room and his chanting has been a cause of annoyance to his roommate. Another way that he connects with his spiritual self is through his music. He brought his guitar into the unit and cherishes playing it. He finds a quiet area of the courtyard and plays. He is finding that the medication is taking away his ability to play music. His hand shakes now and his concentration levels are poor. He says he feels distant and starts to feel sad.

Responding to different values

Depending on the situation we may respond to values in different ways. The following highlights four ways we may respond:

- Ignoring values.
- Shutting down emotions.
- Being blind to values.
- Subsuming values.

Ignoring values

We may manage different values by ignoring them or avoiding situations that demonstrate them and instead choose to be in situations where there are values that are like ours. We choose friends whose values we align with, work in organisations that match our values and enjoy information that reinforces them. We can be taken by surprise when our values are misaligned. You are reading this book according to a choice you made because you value the information in it. This is a straightforward choice: you have read the preamble to the book and consider that it will enrich your knowledge of mental health. If it aligns with your values as well, then you may consider it a very good book. However as you read through it you may possibly realise it is not as significant to you as you thought. There may be certain approaches/beliefs in the book that are at odds with your belief about what is the right approach to mental healthcare. This may be disappointing. You may feel there is nothing about this values difference that you could possibly gain from and you may not finish reading it, close it and put it on your bookshelf and never refer to it again.

You may respond to interpersonal values in the same way and choose to close the conversation and not talk about it. Religion and politics are two such emotive subjects that people may avoid for this reason. This is OK within an equal relationship, but when there is one person who relies on their values being heard and included in order to move forward, then ignoring values is not an option.

Consider Paul's perspective

Paul provides an example of this. From the service's perspective, Paul's chanting is ignored, being understood only for the purpose of judging his mental state. His chanting is seen as a problem. No one asks Paul about his chanting. No one is curious about this significant aspect of Paul. It does not go unnoticed and it is written about in the chart and discussed between the staff in relation to his mental state. A decrease in his chanting is seen as a significant improvement in his mental state. However this is not how Paul views it. Consider the significance of this from Paul's perspective.

Shutting down emotions

Reacting emotionally to values can take us by surprise. Have you ever been in a situation where you have been confronted by another person's values that strongly conflict with your own? It can lead to an argument about what is right, good or bad. I know I have, and my reaction has been powerful. There are certain times in life when we seem to be more susceptible to this. Teenage years are particularly turbulent as we struggle to make sense of our values and have them heard. Childhood years are also emotional times. Maybe you can remember a time as a child when your values were ignored; maybe you were told to eat something that you did not like or go somewhere that you did not want to. As a child, responding emotionally may have been one of your easiest options. As we mature, this type of head-on emotional conflict is rare. However, when you consider the person in the inpatient unit it is maybe not so rare.

Imagine being a patient and faced with a situation where your values are undermined to the point of being told your reality is not right; you are a different person to who you think you are; that you have a mental disorder and need treatment even though you do not think so. Imagine being forced to have treatment against your will.

Imagine being locked up, yet you have not committed a crime and you do not understand why. Imagine the impact that this clash of values could have on you. A clash of values where you believe one thing and everyone else believes something else. Walking away from the situation or ignoring it may not be an option as the whole system reinforces it. You try and reason with the psychiatrist about it, but he does not seem to be listening. Getting into an argument about what you believe is right or wrong, good or bad, is not an option. An emotional reaction can have serious consequences. You have seen what happens to people when they cannot control their emotions; you have heard the panic alarms, seen security being called and people being frogmarched through corridors screaming and shouting. You may feel powerless and forced to conform to someone else's view of reality; you are at your most vulnerable yet have to maintain emotional stability. These conflicts of values are not spoken about. You are trapped according to someone else's ideas.

Consider Jennifer's perspective

Jennifer is part of the team who is looking after Paul. I ask her about Paul's mental state and she reads out the previous day's report.

'Paul has been quiet and co-operative. He has been compliant with all carers. He has spent his day playing his guitar and singing. Generally he appears settled – there is no management problem.'

Paul appears to be emotionally grounded. From a service perspective there is no cause for concern. Would you agree that this is reflective of Paul's situation?

Being blind to values

We work in organisations that function according to agreed values. These are the implicit values that provide the institutional practice or culture of the organisation. Our personal and professional values steer this organisational work. When we are caught up in organisational busyness, we can be blind to the impact of these values on the patient. The values difference is not within our view and unless we actually talk to the patient about their values, we are unaware of them. The power differential that fosters practices of exclusion ensures they are not heard, however this does not mean that they are not there.

Here are some examples:
'I attend appointments but I don't think I have a problem.'
'My voices are seen as problematic yet they have significant meaning for me.'
'I don't like medication yet I am given a depot injection once a fortnight.'
'I am scared that if I don't do as I am told I will end up in seclusion.'
'I don't want to go to the doctor's appointment but you tell me I must.'
'When I disagree with what you say I am told I lack insight.'
'I don't want electric shock treatment but I am made to have it.'

Consider Paul's perspective

What areas do you think we are blind to? Can you think of questions you would ask Paul to find out what his values are?

Subsuming values

One way of closing down values difference is to include them as part of the medical agenda. This can miss the person. Individual difference is placed under a medical umbrella where it is categorised and generalised according to predetermined criteria. The individual difference then becomes a problem to be fixed according to this generalised perspective.

Paul's spirituality is seen as a symptom of his mental disorder. It is seen as a problem. The doctor asks him about it at interview. The conviction he holds around it is seen to be reflective of his mental state.

Consider Paul's perspective

This is Paul's opinion about his spirituality:

'This is something I feel is important for me. When I am in a happy space I am in touch with my spirits and they really help me to get through the day. They are not a problem – they are important for me. They give me strength to carry on. Without them I would be lost.'

Reaching agreement on values

Reasoning through different values involves considered inclusive processes that allow for exploration of different perspectives.

A personal example is that I value living in the countryside and not in the city because I like my personal space but it comes at the expense of travelling long distances to work. My value for space is more important than my value of having less travelling time. But my personal values are not determined in isolation and are considered according to other people involved in the decision to live in the countryside, in this case my family.

Now that my children are getting older, their values of living closer to their school conflicts with my values of living in the countryside. They want to do afterschool activities, they want to be with their friends and they want to be closer to the school. So now I need to consider whether I want to spend time travelling to and from their school or whether I compromise their social activities. My value of providing a social environment for my children now needs consideration.

So I may have to reconsider my values once again. What values are more important for me? My children's social environment or my love of the countryside? But it is not as simple as that – I need to involve other members of the family and consider their perspectives as well. My values will be influenced by them.

I guess that this way of negotiating through situations is something that you will be familiar with. It requires a degree of respect, openness and trust. It is about working out what are the shared values for all concerned and building from there, and ideally it is about coming to consensus where everyone's values are included. The process demonstrates validation by being aware of the problem from the perspective of different values, exploring options, involving the people concerned and negotiating around all perspectives. This process needs to be conducted in a democratic, inclusive and collaborative way to avoid coercion.

Consider Paul's perspective

Flexibility is a mainstay of VBP. What are Paul's values that we could embrace and include?

Disagreeing on values

In order to avoid one set of values dominating another we need to accept that there will be times where values are not agreed on. We need to be able to hold two perspectives to maintain different values when consensus cannot be met.

There may be times when mental illness dominates and enforced action needs to be taken. These are situations where the patient's or another person's life is in jeopardy, where they are suicidal or physically compromised or threatening to harm themselves or others. These situations of extremes need to be acted on. This is the case where situations such as admission under the Mental Health Act demand law-like enforcements which are not in agreement with the person's values.

However this does not mean the person's values should be ignored. Through a process of respect, collaboration and inclusion, the person's values should be kept in play throughout the process of enforcement. Their values continue to drive processes that maintain the connection with the person. Regulating this imbalance by holding both sets of values ensures the person's values are not lost during this time.

The UK Mental Health Act (2008) implementation workbook proposes five codes of practice to bring this about:

1. Least restrictive option and maximising independence.

2. Empowerment and involvement.

3. Respect and dignity.

4. Purpose and effectiveness.

5. Efficiency and equity.

For further information refer to the Care Services Improvement Partnership (CSIP) and The National Institute for Mental Health in England's (2009) *Workbook to Support Implementation of the Mental Health Act 1983 as Amended by the Mental Health Act 2007*.

Consider Paul's perspective

Paul recalls his admission: 'I really didn't know what was happening to me. They brought me into hospital in a police car. I can't remember being told what the reason for this was or if I had time to make sure Jake knew I was OK. It was all a blur for me. I remember the police coming and having to quickly pack a bag then being taken to the unit. I remember people on the street staring and being handcuffed. I really don't know what happened but I remember feeling scared.'

Write an alternative script for Paul's admission under the MHA from a VBP perspective.

Tips to engage with the patient's values

- Get to know the person and what is important for them.
- Make the patient's values central to your plan.
- Talk about and include the patient's values in the team review.
- Check in and confirm your understanding.
- Be dynamic.
- Consider your pre-judgements.
- Be mindful of maintaining a balance of patient values and medical knowledge.

Section 6: How to manage your values to keep the person central

Skill: knowledge

Considering your values

Your values play an integral role in a VBP approach. Your values are seen through the choices you make. The decisions and care you deliver accords as much with your values as they do with the patient's. Here are some examples of clinical choices that demonstrate this.

- You ask the patient to leave the group session to see the doctor.
- You walk past the patient sitting in the foyer but acknowledge the staff member and ask them how their day has been.
- You go across to the coffee shop and ask the patient you are looking after if they would like a coffee.
- You work afternoon shifts rather than morning shifts because you have to take the children to school.

We are all different; we have different ideas about what is good or bad, right or wrong. On the big ticket items we tend to reach consensus on what is good or bad, for example murdering another person is bad, genocide is bad, pain is bad. But when it comes to the little ticket items, our preferences may not be so easily shared.

> **Thinking activity:**
> What are your values? What is important for you?
> What makes a good day at work?

How values influence different clinical decisions

Different people have different values and will act according to their values in different ways. For example:

> **Case example**
> The morning shift starts at 7am.
> When Gordon is on shift he makes sure all the patients are given their medication early, even if it means waking them up in the morning.
> When Jenny is on shift she usually gives the morning medication after breakfast and allows patients a two hour time frame.
> When Robert is on shift he leaves the patients to sleep and gives them their medication when they wake up.
> Here we have three staff members with different approaches to medication. Their degree of flexibility reflects their view of what is right or wrong practice according to their set of values. Rules are bent and situations amended to fit in with these values.
> This situation of different values can be a problem for the patient on the receiving end if their values are not considered. The patient Paul feels as if he has been left out of the loop.
> Here is his response:
> *'When Gordon is on shift I don't get a lie-in. When Robert is on I sleep in. Most of the time I don't mind getting up, but there have been times when I would have liked to sleep in; you know when I have been up late for whatever reason and there is no group meeting or reason for me to get up at 7am. I really don't understand why they can't leave my medication for a couple of hours – I never take it at this time when I am at home.'*

As this example demonstrates, values are shown by what we do; the action we take. Whether these values are a problem or not depends on how they fit with other values.

Accepting values difference

Your values agenda is determined by your professional, organisational and personal values. Using these alone, without the patient's perspective, can lead to a values agenda that is more centred on meeting your needs than the patient's. The extreme of this was seen in the case of institutional practice. To avoid this, the patient's perspective needs to be central to clinical decisions. You may find that you do not agree with the patient's values as they conflict with yours. Being aware of this, tolerating this difference and negotiating alternative options, rather than controlling values difference, is important if token VBP is to be avoided. Putting the patient agenda at the centre may mean that your values are compromised. However, if you see it from a person-centred practice perspective, then your values will support, not control the patient's values. The following provides examples of this. It is split into organisational, personal and professional values and demonstrates examples of where these get in the way of providing person-centred care.

Personal values

It is important to be aware of your personal values, as they will influence the decisions you make on a daily basis. Think about your role, the choices you make and situations when your personal values may get in the way. What happens when you have a 'bad day', how do you manage?

Consider the following scenario.

Case example

It is Tuesday morning and the breakfast trolley has arrived. The trolley is sent from the kitchen with pre-prepared breakfasts allocated to each patient.

It is busy in the dining room as always, but particularly as today as it is the day for electroconvulsive therapy treatment (ECT). Security is present, standing at the back of the dining room waiting to escort a couple of the patients who are going for ECT.

Janice is the nursing assistant helping patients to get their breakfast from the trolley.

There is a spillage of water on the floor from one of the elderly patients.

A patient named Sarah shouts out to Janice, *'Hey you need to clean the floor; someone could slip.'*

Janice responds, *'This is not my job; get a cloth and do it yourself.'*

Continued

> *Case example continued*
>
> Sarah replies, *'I don't get paid; you do; you clean it up and get those lousy security guards out of here they shouldn't be in here watching us like coppers; you go and annoy somebody else.'*
> Janice shouts across the dining room, *'Don't you talk like that.'*
> Sarah replies, *'We don't have coppers in here; scum; go find another innocent to hassle.'*
> Janice says, *'If you can't stop shouting you will need to leave.'*
> Sarah says, *'Yes, and what you going to do about it, you the lazy arse that can't even clean the mess up on the floor.'*
> Janice says, *'It's not my job to clean up water, you do it and shut your mouth or you'll end up going to HDU [High Dependency Unit].'*
> At which point, Sarah stood up.

What could be contributing to Sarah and Janice's reactions? The way we would know the answers to these questions is by knowing their values. Janice was having a bad day; there is a lot going on in her life at the moment. Sarah has had traumatic interactions with the police in the past.

Consider times when your personal values have been voiced. For example, I may shout and get annoyed at the person in the shopping centre that walks in front of me and nearly knocks me over, but I would not do that to the person in the inpatient unit who is running to get to the door to greet his visitor. I may get angry at my son who leaves the milk on the side rather than putting it back in the fridge, but I wouldn't get angry at the patient who leaves the milk out.

What's the difference? Why am I more tolerant of one then the other? What am I doing with my personal values when I am at work?

Organisational values

Healthcare organisations have patient's health and well-being as their priority. They determine and monitor practice through standards and quality agendas. These are fed into the work area through policies and procedures. Organisations also deliver services that are inclusive, respectful and person centred. Including values such as respect, autonomy, integrity, and caring for people within these is required if the fundamental goal of person-centred care is to be achieved.

In the UK the National Health Service Institute for Innovation and Improvement has developed a set of 11 resources from the Living Our Local Values Project (Department of Health, 2009). These are:

1. Getting started.
2. Value of values.
3. Defining and refreshing our values.
4. How we behave with our partners.
5. How we behave with our patients.
6. How we behave with each other.
7. How we communicate.
8. Our decision making.
9. Our leadership.
10. Our organisational process.
11. How to assess impact.

They are available for download from the following site: http://www.institute.nhs.uk/building_capability/living_our_local_values/resources.html
The rule-like policies and procedures provide the greatest good to the greatest number, whereas the values agenda reflects individual perspectives. When individual and organisational agendas align there is no problem, however sticking rigidly to policies when they don't align (due to individual differences) may result in abuse.

Case example: Keith

It is 1:30pm on Tuesday afternoon in the inpatient unit and Mary is the nurse in charge. The day has been uneventful; busy but nothing unusual. Jason is the recreation officer in the High Dependency Unit (HDU).

Keith has been a patient in the HDU for a few days. He is told that his brother is here to visit and has brought his nephew Joel with him. Keith is very fond of his nephew and they are very close.

Visiting time on the unit is 3pm until 5pm. This has been found to be the best time because it is outside meal times, doctors' visiting time and change of shift times.

The nurse in charge told Keith that he could not see his nephew because it was outside visiting time. Jason, the recreation officer, volunteered to spend extra time in the unit to sit with Keith's nephew and be around during his visit. His brother asked the nurse to make a special allowance and explained the situation. Mary reiterated to Keith that there was no visiting allowed at that time. Nursing handover took place from 2:30pm and 3:00pm and all the nurses were busy from lunch time up until after the handover. There were no nursing staff available to assist with visiting at this time and he would have to go away and come back at 3pm. Unfortunately this was not an option as Joel had to leave by 3pm.

Organisational rational for visiting times

The rules of visiting times derive from organisational consideration for what is best for patients. That is the safest time when most staff are around and there is minimal impact on medical treatments.

The dilemma

This stems from a person who cannot keep to these rules because of their particular circumstances. As was discussed in Section 2, when rules dictate, individual needs can be lost. By ignoring the person's values we are not meeting the ethical principles of doing good. This is only done by including the person's values.

Options

The solution is to find flexible ways that support the inclusion of the individual difference that the person brings to the situation. One of the options in Keith's situation would be to involve the recreation officer or a nurse from another area. Maybe the handover could be completed later.

Professional values

There are times when professional knowledge can get in the way of seeing the person. The following is an example where the patient's behaviour is viewed according to a pathological diagnosis which shuts down any explorative discourse. As a result, the process of decision making was not patient inclusive. According to ethical principles, the doctor is doing the right thing; he is working within his scope of practice and has an agreed professional diagnosis to determine his decision. However, without due consideration for the patient's perspective (particularly the changes that result from the patient's situation) the process of making the decision seems flawed.

This scenario paints a picture between risk and autonomy. It is filled with different values messages. What messages are you hearing?

Case example: Mira

Mira is a 30-year-old woman who has been in the inpatient unit for two weeks.

Mira had made a plan to leave the unit to go across the road to pay her electricity bill but was stopped on her way out by Dr John and questioned as to where she was going. On hearing that she was going across the road, Dr John asked her not to leave the unit, that she was not well enough and she needed to go back onto the ward. Mira was angry at hearing this and let her frustrations out by shouting, going to her bedroom and slamming the door. Dr John followed her to her room but she refused to let him in, shouting abuse through the locked door. He informed Mira through the closed bedroom door to calm down and instructed the junior doctors to give her 150mg of Acuphase and seclusion if necessary.

Mira's nurse Simone was requested by the junior doctor to give her the Acuphase (Acuphase is a long acting anti-psychotic that lasts for about three days). Simone started to draw up the medication. She did not agree and perceived it as a drastic response to an understandably frustrating situation. However she was going to give it to the patient because it was something that the doctor had prescribed.

The doctors had now left the area and gone back to their rooms.

Mira had left her bedroom and was in the court area. A senior nurse who had been witness to the situation caught up with her and asked her how she was now doing and that she was going to be given Acuphase. Mira said she would settle down in time and told her that she should not have shouted like that at the doctor but she needed to pay her electricity bill otherwise it would be cut off and she would have to pay to have it turned on again. She said she really did not want any medication that was going to knock her out for three days. She was having her daughter visit that afternoon and she wanted to speak to the doctor to apologise for her behaviour.

The senior nurse returned to the doctor who was now in his room and enquired as to what had happened. He told her that Mira was unwell; she was attempting to leave the ward. The nurse informed him that the situation had now changed that she was in the court area and requesting not to have the injection. At which point he said she should have the injection, that she had bipolar disorder and she was labile and dangerous and that her screaming behaviour was testimony to this.

Mira was given the injection.

Conclusion

This guide has been a journey through an awareness, reasoning, communication and knowledge of values and how to work with them to provide person-centred care. The fundamental message throughout the guide has been on tolerating rather than controlling different values.

Talking about values and being open to difference as a potential positive attribute for patient well-being is necessary if dominance of one set of values over another is to be avoided. Engaging with the person's values supports a trusting and respectful relationship. Using the relationship to cajole or coerce the person to meet medical agendas is not part of VBP. Rather, VBP supports different values for the understanding they bring, to enrich medical understanding according to this difference and to support a relationship based on mutual respect.

References

Beauchamp TL & Childress JF (1994) *Principles of Biomedical Ethics* (4th edition) Oxford: Oxford University Press.

Care Services Improvement Partnership (CSIP) and The National Institute for Mental Health in England (NIMHE) (2008) *Workbook to Support Implementation of the Mental Health Act 1983 as Amended by the Mental Health Act 2007*. London: Department of Health.

Deegan P (1992) The independent living movement and people with psychiatric disabilities: taking back control over our own lives. *Psychosocial Rehabilitation Journal* **15** (3) 12.

Department of Health (2009) *Living our Local Values*. NHS Institute for Innovation and Improvement. Available at: http://www.institute.nhs.uk/building_capability/living_our_local_values/resources.html (accessed May 2016).

Faulkner A (2005) Institutional conflict: the state of play in adult acute psychiatric wards. *The Journal of Adult Protection* **7** (4) 6–12

Fulford KWM (2004) Facts/values: ten principles of values-based medicine. In: J Radden (Ed.) *The Philosophy of Psychiatry: A companion* (pp205–234). New York: Oxford University Press.

Hawksworth W (2016) *Applying Values-based Practice for People Experiencing Psychosis: A training pack for inpatient settings*. Brighton: Pavilion Publishing.

The Health Foundation (2014) *Person Centred Care Made Simple* [online]. Available at: http://personcentredcare.health.org.uk/ (accessed April 2016).

Woodbridge K & Fulford KWM (2004) *Whose Values? A workbook for values-based practice in mental healthcare* [online]. The Sainsbury Centre for Mental Health. Available at: www.valuesbasedpractice.org (accessed April 2016).

Additional resources

Theory guides

Fulford KWM, Peile E & Carroll H (2012) *Essential Values-Based Practice: Clinical stories linking science with people.* Cambridge: Cambridge University Press.

Loughlin M (2014) *Debates in Values-Based Practice: Arguments for and against.* Cambridge: Cambridge University Press.

Slade M (2009) *Personal Recovery and Mental Illness: A guide for mental health professionals.* Cambridge: Cambridge University Press.

Thistlethwaite JE (2012) *Values-based Interprofessional Collaborative Practice: Working together in healthcare.* Cambridge: Cambridge University Press.

Online

CSIP/NIMHE (2008) *3 Keys to a Shared Approach in Mental Health Assessment.* London: DoH. Available at: www.valuesbasedpractice.org
The 10 Essential Shared Capabilities to Support Person-centred Care. Edinburgh: NHS. Available at: www.nes.scot.nhs.uk/media/351385/10_essential_shared_capabilities_2011.pdf

Whose Values? A workbook for Values-Based Practice in Mental Healthcare. London: The Sainsbury Centre for Mental Health. Available at: www.valuesbasedpractice.org

More about VBP
www.valuesbasedpractice.org

To get involved

The Collaborating Centre for Values-based Practice:
www.valuesbasedpractice.org

Mental health charities

SANE: www.sane.org
Rethink Mental Illness: www.rethink.org
Mental Health Foundation: www.mentalhealth.org.uk

Appendix

Ten principles for VBP
(Woodbridge & Fulford, 2004)

Practice skills
1. Awareness: of the values present in a given situation. Careful attention to language is one way of raising awareness of values.

2. Reasoning: using a clear reasoning process to explore the values present when making decisions.

3. Knowledge: of the values and facts relevant to the specific situation.

4. Communication: combined with the previous three skills, this is central to the resolution of conflicts and the decision making process.

Models of service delivery
5. User-centred: the first source of information on values in any situation is the perspective of the service user concerned.

6. Multidisciplinary: conflicts of values are not resolved in values-based practice by applying a 'pre-prescribed rule', but by working towards a balance of different perspectives (e.g. multidisciplinary team working together).

Values-based practice and evidence-based practice
7. The 'two feet' principle: all decisions are based on facts and values (values base and evidence base work together).

8. The 'squeaky wheel principle': we only notice values when there is a problem.

9. Science and values: increasing scientific knowledge creates choice in healthcare, which introduces wide differences in values.

Partnership
10. Partnership: in values-based practice decisions are taken by service users and the providers of care working in partnership.